Chronic Fatigue Syndrome, ME and Fibromyalgia – The Long Awaited Cure.

Dr David Mickel MBChB MRCGP
Founder of Mickel Health Initiatives Ltd

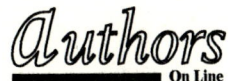

Visit us online at www.authorsonline.co.uk

An AuthorsOnLine Book

Copyright © Authors OnLine Ltd 2004

Text Copyright © Dr David Mickel 2004

Cover design by James Fitt and Sandra Davis ©

All rights reserved. No part of this publication may be reproduced, stored in a retrieval system, or transmitted in any form or by any means, electronic, mechanical, photocopy, recording or otherwise, without prior written permission of the copyright owner. Nor can it be circulated in any form of binding or cover other than that in which it is published and without similar condition including this condition being imposed on a subsequent purchaser.

ISBN 0 7552 0143 4

Authors OnLine Ltd
40 Castle Street
Hertford SG14 1HR
England

This book is also available in e-book format, details of which are available at www.authorsonline.co.uk

Contents

Introduction	1
Chapter 1- The Road to Discovery	4
Chapter 2 – Underlying Concepts	12
Chapter 3 – 'E-motions' – The Truth Revealed	18
Chapter 4 – A Theory of Vibration	23
Chapter 5- Cellular Memory	28
Chapter 6 – So What Are Symptoms?	33
Chapter 7- Chronic Fatigue Syndrome, ME and Fibromyalgia	37
Chapter 8 – The Condition of 'Hypothalamitis'	40
Chapter 9 - This is NOT Depression!	52
Chapter 10 – Mickel Therapy Treatment – What to expect.	53
Chapter 11 – Testimonials	55
Appendix – Contact Details	68

Introduction

The purpose of this book is to share my findings in treating the conditions of Chronic Fatigue Syndrome, ME and Fibromyalgia. The result of the treatment is very exciting and will bring hope to the many who suffer these conditions. I am hopeful that what is written in the following will be informative to sufferers, their family and professionals alike. A great deal of scepticism and misleading information has been written in this field and I am hopeful that at least some of this can be put to rest.

Unfortunately this book has had to be rewritten and I would like to explain the reasons behind this. When I first found a treatment process that was consistently curing individuals, in May 2001, I decided to share this exciting news with my friend and colleague Dr John Eaton. Dr Eaton was my trainer during my years of learning about Ericksonian Hypnotherapy and taught me many things that helped me find the successful treatment for CFS/ME and Fibromyalgia. I therefore chose to share this knowledge with him and we went onto form the limited company Reverse Therapy Ltd.

Our mission statement was simple:

"To eradicate Chronic Fatigue Syndrome/ME and Fibromyalgia and to teach others how to do it"

However, our alliance did not work out and we have since gone our separate ways. An unfortunate side effect of this was that the jointly written book on Reverse Therapy treatment could not be published. I have therefore rewritten it in my own way. This has actually not been a negative thing in the long run since it has given me the opportunity to review its content and update it to contain some of the things that have evolved in my own delivery of the treatment now known as Mickel Therapy.

There is a full spectrum of these illnesses from a bedridden state of horrendous suffering to a frustrating life of low energy and sub-optimal physical and mental performance. Considering there are more than 400,000 sufferers in the UK alone and little help available other than at best palliative treatments, Mickel Therapy is very pleased now to be able to alleviate such suffering.

I am confident this book will bring some hope to sufferers and a sense of light at the end of the tunnel. Unfortunately much of the last couple of decades of research has done little to achieve it and this is principally because it has been directed at looking at effects rather than getting to the root cause.

This includes expensive and fruitless investigations of complicated and detailed muscular metabolism, immune system analysis, viral titres and a long list of others that merely investigate effects and do not focus on cause.

The root cause in my opinion is a dysfunctional Hypothalamus gland (I have called 'Hypothalamitis') and I am confident my treatment has found a solution to this physical problem. This however creates further scepticism towards my claim that we can cure these conditions. People quite rightly ask, "But how can a talking treatment cure a physical condition?" I am hopeful this book will go a long way to explaining this.

Bearing in mind that the concentration of most sufferers is impaired I have tried to keep the chapters in the book short and easily understandable without losing necessary theory. However should the reader have further need for detail then they can contact Mickel Therapy using the details in the Appendix at the end of this book.

This book will look at the conditions from a new perspective while hopefully dispelling some of the mystery surrounding them. While not designed to teach the process, it will certainly help people who decide to take the treatment to get started much more easily while also helping those interested in training to make an informed decision about this.

Chapter 1

The Road to Discovery

My Story

I sometimes reflect on my journey through life and wonder at the decisions I made and how they came about - none more so than my choice of career to become a Doctor and then a Therapist.

I enjoyed a good secondary school education without ever considering what I was going to do when 'I grew up'. I had contemplated Veterinary Medicine but this was probably more due to a romantic interest in the James Herriot novels than any real vocational drive. The thought of training to become a Doctor did not ever cross my mind until I was ready to leave school - it took me by surprise as much as it did my family. I remember clearly the day the University application forms were to be returned. I was sitting at the kitchen table throwing different course suggestions into the room at my mother who was now becoming tired of being my sounding board. 'French and zoology? French and business? Law …or what about…..?' Then it happened. I heard or rather felt the answer coming from deep inside me – Medicine! Where that came from I was not sure. I have developed many beliefs since this time and I now know this was what people would term 'my calling'. It pervaded my whole being and though Medicine had never crossed my mind before this moment, I knew my decision had been made there and then.

Still slightly bemused at my own decision I headed to Aberdeen to start my studies in Medicine at the University there. I spent a fruitless year trying to find 'My Self' but instead found myself red faced in front of the Dean and his Board of advisors trying to persuade them to let me back into the Faculty, having messed up my first exams. As fate would have it, they agreed to let me try again and eventually I completed my studies with no further hiccups.

The world of Medicine was fascinating to me and I took well to my various hospital jobs and the responsibilities that came with them. The 100 hours plus per week were bearable due to the interest I had in learning about physical diseases and the advanced treatments there to deal with them. I eventually decided to venture into General Practice and following a couple of years as an itinerant Locum Doctor I found a Practice in Elgin in the North of Scotland.

My initial enjoyment in General Practice was high. The hours were long and the paperwork barely tolerable but it was a privileged role. I was at the centre of family life dealing with the physical, mental and social disorders people experience from birth to death. This was both very challenging and rewarding - but something didn't feel right about the orthodox medical approach to healthcare. My days were spent prescribing medication for conditions and then counter prescribing to help ease the problems caused by side effects associated with the first medication – this became a never-ending spiral. Leaving aside all the political issues that filled me with frustration and despair, I was beginning to realize there had to be more to the promotion of health, the causes of illness and how we should treat them.

I began to get interested in alternative or complimentary health approaches. I read copious books on acupuncture, homeopathy, herbal medicine, Ayurveda, Reiki, hypnosis, and much about Spiritual healing. My bookshelves were sagging with a vast array of esoteric literature, much to the amusement of my fellow doctors. My intention was to broaden my knowledge and allow myself to feel more comfortable in my role as GP but the opposite happened.

Gathering knowledge and interests in these subjects merely served to fuel my growing discontent with conventional medicine and the part I played in delivering it. Some may say I grew a conscience. I was aware that most of the drugs I prescribed were alien compounds whose side effects stretched to pages and pages. Moreover, many of them simply masked the symptoms of the illness, rather than addressing the deeper causes of ill health.

It was at this time I started to look into training in psychotherapy. Again I had never contemplated such a thing and it appeared to come out of nowhere. On reflection, I can see this was similar to the 'calling' I got to do Medicine, not premeditated but completely out of the blue. The decision happened overnight and before I knew it I had enrolled into a school in London to study Ericksonian techniques. I completed the two-year diploma course and began to see people in my spare time. Before long I had a large private clinic which required me to cut back on my time in General Practice. As I continued to work in my new field I started to get the answers to my questions about General Practice and why it did not feel comfortable. Medical training had taught me to isolate symptoms and organize them into systems of disease: respiratory, gastrointestinal, nervous etc. I began to realize that this model of thinking served to split the individual into parts not representative of the whole. I soon became interested in the more holistic approach of mind-body medicine. This made much more sense to me and I became acutely aware of changes in my practice both in Medicine and Therapy. I soon began to consider the health problems of my clients and patients from a different perspective. On the one hand this was very exciting but on the other it lead to frustrations in my General Practice role as the system was not set up for this kind of work. Indeed it was more like trying to provide health care to patients whizzing past on a conveyor belt with a maximum of 10 minutes allocated to each one.

My times spent doing therapy soon became the most enjoyable aspect of my working life to date. I was beginning to see the potential of a mind-body perspective and the successful way this could help with problems that previously I had only had a prescription pad to turn to. It was during this time I started to come across the conditions Chronic Fatigue Syndrome/ME and Fibromyalgia in the therapy room. I had of course had experience of these in General Practice but other than offering a supportive shoulder I had very little to offer. Like my colleagues, I was at a loss as to how to explain these illnesses. The routine tests that doctors depend on to help in diagnosis, were usually borderline or normal. It wasn't long before I found myself falling into the trap of thinking the symptoms must be due to a depressive illness. Fortunately, fate had other plans for me and I began a relationship with a previously healthy and vivacious, young woman whose whole life had been turned on it's head when she developed 'ME'.

The two years that followed, with Sally, were a turning point for me as a Doctor in my understanding of this condition. Like many people with her condition it had been suggested to her she may have 'Depression' but there was no doubt in my mind this loving, happy person was as far from being depressed as I was. The bottom line was that she was completely and utterly exhausted. Her other symptoms of aches, pains, headaches and general malaise were very real and through time I soon learned to recognise the external signs. This was not the effect of Depression. Any lowering of her mood was understandable considering the degree of suffering she was enduring.

It is difficult for me to find the words to express the frustration I felt as a helpless partner and more importantly a Doctor whose chosen vocation was to improve the health of people in need. To watch the brave fight she had daily with her physical state was inspiring. Here was someone who had always been very physically active and mentally active now reduced to survival instincts only. As well as my acute sense of frustration I had to admit to admiring her ability to get up each day to cope with unimaginable discomfort and despair. In reflection I know it was the strength of these feelings and the experiences we shared during our relationship that led me to commit to understanding these conditions and find a way to treating them successfully.

Over the following years I started to see more people with CFS/ME and Fibromyalgia in my role as therapist. I knew successes in this field where few and far between. I felt this was due to the fact that we did not know what was really going wrong within the person presenting. After all, how do you fix a fault when you don't know where or what it is? I had a good basic training in therapeutic techniques and was perhaps what would be known as an eclectic therapist. I started to try a variety of techniques to deal with these challenging cases. Initially these were frustrating times and any improvements were limited and not up to my self-imposed high standards.

Over the following two years I worked tirelessly with CFS/ME and Fibromyalgia cases. Through trial and error I developed a successful therapeutic process. I was delighted to see consistent 100% recovery in all cases completing treatment regardless of duration or severity of illness. It was following the treatment of one certain case that I decided to leave General Practice and commit to body-mind medicine. The client in question had had Fibromyalgia for 42 years! The degree of suffering she endured was terrible with daily pain and weakness in her arms and legs it was a wonder that she did not go to her bed and never get up. I will always remember the day she came in for her appointment and began to cry. Inwardly I was ready to be disappointed that she was feeling no better when she told me that she had been completely symptom free for the last two weeks! I could feel the tears well up in my own eyes and in a flash it became clear to me that I could no longer justify my comfortable salary and position as General Practitioner while people like this were suffering. Again, on reflection I recognize that my inner voice increased the volume on 'my calling' and clarity followed. That night I wrote the hardest letter of my life and the next day handed in my resignation to my General Practice. My attention was now fully on the treatment of Chronic Fatigue Syndrome, ME and Fibromyalgia.

Turning Point

Having tried to treat the many cases that came my way in private practice using my Ericksonian therapy training, Neurolinguistic Programming (NLP) and even Cognitive Behavioural Therapy I started to doubt my abilities. This frustration was my biggest challenge to date and I came very close to packing it all in. Then I reviewed some of the principles that the genius therapist Milton Erickson had founded. In short this led me to view symptoms of any illness differently. Namely Erickson believed symptoms were 'solutions' and therefore should be utilized and not resisted. As I will discuss in later chapters this is a very different and challenging attitude to symptoms, whereby symptoms need to be welcomed and viewed as wisdom to be learned from. In Erickson's terms this wisdom was generated by the unconscious mind and indeed I referred in early cases to this distinction between unconscious and conscious mind until I settled on the terms 'body-mind' and 'head-mind' respectively. These terms will be explained in more detail in subsequent chapters.

This shift in my approach started to rekindle my interest and hopes in success. Throughout 2000-1 I was now the crazy doctor who thought that symptoms were not to be gotten rid of but rather welcomed, interpreted and translated in order to discover what wisdom they offered. These were interesting and challenging times considering my medical training as I attempted to put aside my reflex medical trained reaction to get rid of symptoms of illness quickly. I can't say how glad I am that I stuck with it.

To give you an idea of what type of insanity went on in my consulting room I can give you an example from one of my earliest cases which took place in early 2000. The scene is set for Mike to come for his second session. He was suffering from a three year, history of Chronic Fatigue Syndrome:

Dr M : " Hi Mike, please come in and sit down. Now then have you had any symptoms sent by your unconscious mind for us to look at?"
Mike : " What? Dae ye mean have I been ill, like?"
Dr M : "Well...er...sort of. Do you remember we spoke last time about how your symptoms were actually wisdom sent by your unconscious mind for us to receive and translate?"
Mike : "Aye...I think so?"
Dr M : " Okay so have you had a lot of symptoms since I last saw you?"
Mike : "Aye, loads of them all the time"

At this point I made a critical over-estimate of Mike's understanding of the theory I had tried to explain to him and I said something that, the minute it left my mouth, I instantly regretted - especially seeing as although fatigued Mike was built like an African bull elephant...

Dr M : " Oh excellent! That's good"
Mike : " Good!? Good!? What the *****************"

As Mike leapt to his feet and angrily headed to the door, using words I had not heard used since school days and many new ones besides, I realised all too late the difficulties of getting my clients to understand this new concept. I had learned a tough lesson and it is down to Mike as to why I put so much effort into learning to deliver what is now Mickel Therapy in a way that all clients could understand and partake in. I hope the following chapters will make this process even easier for any of you that do decide to embark on treatment with Mickel Therapy.

(I am glad to say Mike returned and is now symptom free).

Chapter 2

Underlying concepts

Understanding the underlying concepts of this therapy will make receiving and successfully completing it much easier. Indeed from analysis of my cases the point where the treatment process speeds to a successful end is directly related to the time where this 'penny drops'. I will endeavour in the following chapters to make this easier for readers of all ages and professional backgrounds. Many may find the content of this a challenge to their current understanding - I empathise fully with you, I also had to challenge my pre-existing beliefs about health and 'dis-ease'.

Let's first look at a concise list of the concepts involved in the theory:

- **CFS/ME and Fibromyalgia are caused by a dysfunction of the hypothalamus gland** - subsequent chapters should make this a very reasonable assumption to make.
- **Body-Mind (Body) has an inherent intelligence that exists at a cellular level** - please see text below on 'e-motions', symptoms as communication and State Dependant Memory.
- **Symptoms, although often uncomfortable are helpful and necessary communication from the body-mind.**
- **Psychosomatic illness is a nonsensical term when looked at through Mickel Therapy eyes** - this implies the psyche (head-mind) has the ability to create 'dis-ease' and symptoms of this. As we will discuss this is not the case.
- **Once Symptoms are interpreted, translated and responded to appropriately they are no longer produced** - this is the concept I struggled with so

long until it has now proven itself over and over again.
- **CFS/ME and Fibromyalgia are not cause by viral infections** - such infections are effects of 'Hypothalamitis' state on the immune function and **not** the cause.
- **CFS/ME and Fibromyalgia are NOT examples of Depression** - Please see relevant chapter.

These concepts are accepted more readily by some clients than others and this is understandable, given our Western cultural upbringings and education. It is however a fact that all the clients that have been cured over the last few years have accepted this at some level or otherwise not allowed any doubts to halt their treatment process. Readers are strongly encouraged to check with their own 'body-mind' on completion of this book whether it feels acceptable to them. Further clarification can be obtained through the website if necessary - details in Appendix.

'Being in two minds'

This is the poorly understood nature of a human's existence - we live perpetually in 'two minds'. Surely this can't be healthy - indeed there is plenty of evidence to support the fact that it is **not** and that this phenomenon creates 'dis-ease' on a regular basis. From my point of view this is the crux of all illness. In order to understand this bold statement let's take a closer look at these two minds.
These could be what Milton Erickson and others have referred to as unconscious and conscious mind but we now introduce them as body-mind (The Body) and head-mind (Head).

Introduction to 'The Body'

As previously referred to, there are numerous names that could be given to what we refer to as the body-mind or 'body'. This term has been chosen to 'fit best' with different ethnic and religious backgrounds in order to make the delivery of therapy easier. However it should be kept in mind, you might have other terms of reference you are more comfortable with and your therapists will be able to adapt accordingly if necessary. The most important realisation to take on board is that there are definitely two separate intelligences within each of us.

The 'body' therefore represents the body-mind, unconscious mind, inner voice, inner being, heart, possibly soul and many other labels. Regardless of what we call this intelligence it has the same qualities and plays the same role in the human existence. This is namely to keep us safe in an unpredictable world. People often ask me where this intelligence is. This is a testing question and I, in all honesty, am not sure. However I would imagine it is in every cell of our body, all around us and possibly more concentrated in the solar plexus area, thus explaining what is known as gut feelings.

The 'body' is therefore:

- ♦ An intelligent source of wisdom
- ♦ Protective of the self
- ♦ Omniscient
- ♦ Authentic and will not lie
- ♦ Constantly aware of the world in which it exists
- ♦ The source of our true nature - 'soul/personality'
- ♦ Responsible for remembering all that is important to remember - which as we will see it does by using State Dependant or chemical memory at a cellular level.

- **'The Boss!'**

In short the body's job is to protect the Self. It does this by continually evaluating the world it finds itself in and then communicates its feedback in the form of truthful e-motions or feelings that can be felt as physical symptoms. We will look in more detail at this in subsequent chapters.

Unfortunately this protective role often fails to get through to us and this results in 'dis-ease' as we will discuss in the course of this book. We are very practised at missing this communication from our bodies. Indeed cultural and societal pressures in the Western world are still such that they lead us further from our body's intelligence. It is little wonder there is such evidence of 'dis-ease' throughout the Western world. Through Mickel Therapy we are dedicated to correcting this.

A Few words about the 'head'

I now understand why my early attempts to treat cases of CFS/ME and Fibromyalgia were doomed to failure. I was employing classical psychotherapeutic principles which are basically designed to treat 'head-mind'. This was never going to succeed because the conditions are not psychological, but physical and therefore arise within the 'body' and not the psyche. This is why the application of treatments such as CBT as suggested by current medical wisdom is both frustrating and disrespectful of the conditions true nature.

Mickel Therapy focuses solely on the body-mind (body) intelligence and pays no reference to the head or 'head-mind', which is more than adequately attended to by these conventional psychotherapies. But it is worth understanding the 'nature of this beast'.

Conventional wisdom perceives the head as the 'mind' and

therefore the supreme intelligence. Mickel Therapists realise this is simply **not** the case. This explains why such approaches do not resolve the underlying need for the symptoms of 'dis-ease' and they are likely to continue to manifest.

So where does this head intelligence fit into the picture we are creating?

Well, firstly the head could otherwise be known as the conscious mind, brain or chatter box. In health it is imperative that it is guided by the wisdom of the body and not be allowed to over-ride or distort the information the 'body' sends. Unfortunately this is rarely the case. Human 'dis-ease' occurs when the head acts like an unruly employee who does not follow the boss's instructions. As Mickel Therapists our job is to 'reverse' this unhealthy state of affairs - **not** by doing any 'head work' but rather by empowering the body and allowing it to do its job - namely communicating its needs for a healthy interaction with our world.

Fortunately as we apply the Mickel Therapy principles, this disruptive influence of the 'head' soon ceases and the two intelligences of 'body' and 'head' start to work hand in hand as a team. It is at this stage that health can be enjoyed. So in other words the following salient points become obvious:

In 'dis-ease' the head:

- Does not align its thoughts with the body's intelligence
- Magnifies and distorts 'e-motions' from the body
- Misrepresents 'truth'
- Encourages actions that do not agree with the body's intelligence

- Removes us from our true nature and authentic self
- Tries to take over as **'The Boss'**

In health the head:

- Aligns its thinking with the body's intelligence
- Accepts the body's e-motional evaluations
- Works with the body to face and deal with the truth
- Generates actions that are in accordance with the body's intelligence
- Allows the body to manifest the true nature of the self.

In this way the truth most definitely sets us free.

Chapter 3

'E-motions' – the truth revealed.

It was with difficulty that I personally came to the realisation that all that I had been taught about emotions was wrong. From a psychological point of view these are thought to be the result of our thoughts and we are encouraged to look upon them as unwanted and often wrong. This basic understanding was soon shattered as my experience of cases grew. This assumes the emotions are created according to what our 'head-mind' (head) thinks and conventional treatments are designed to correct this. Tools such as affirmations, CBT, counselling and psychotherapy aim to alter how we feel by working with the 'head'. This is based on a wrong assumption - that is - that our emotions or feelings are caused by the head's opinions. This is simply **not** true and it is for this reason that Mickel Therapy agrees with the more accurate term 'e-motion' or translated 'energy-in–motion'. We will look at this in more detail below.

So what are these pesky waves in our tranquil lake of happiness? Well, the good news is that they must always be **useful** and **necessary** communications from our body - if somewhat uncomfortable occasionally. It would be inconceivable to imagine that our body would ever wish us any harm, considering that it is part of us and has a large investment in our well being.

Emotions or as we prefer to call them, 'e-motions' are **'energy-in-motion'.** In simple terms, they are the energy of situations transduced by the body into the energy of 'e-motion' that reflect the body's evaluation of these situations and **not** the head. The head's role comes in after this energy is created as a feeling and at this point it can distort or magnify their inherent truthful assessment. This then leads to psychological states that conventional therapies attempt to correct.

Creation of 'E-motions'

The following describes how these communications from our body intelligence are created.

Figure 1

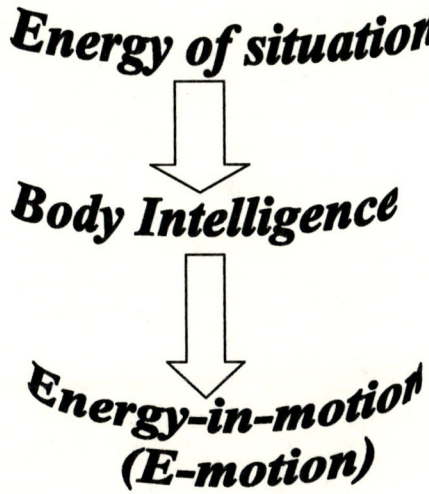

In order to understand the inherent principle shown in *Figure 1*, we have to view matter in a slightly different way. In order to avoid going into hefty detail of which I am no expert, readers with an interest to do so are encouraged to read "Quantum Healing" by Deepak Chopra MD.

So let's look at some of the concepts involved in Quantum Physics. Put simply this branch of science has began to break down and examine the building blocks of all matter and indeed 'non-matter' such as gases. As cells, atoms and smaller building blocks are broken down we start to arrive at the startling understanding that all things are actually made of a 'non-solid' energy. It is according to the frequency at which this energy vibrates that denotes what it becomes in solid form. For example if my human brain were able to process the information around me then I would see no solid matter but rather a massive swirling interaction of different colours of light energy. Now I appreciate this is getting into the realms of 'beam me up Scotty!' But perhaps science is actually getting nearer being able to control the energy of matter in order for us to consider transportation to the 'Starship Enterprise' - but this is a separate discussion.

Getting back to the creation of 'e-motions' - what does this all mean? Well, in simple terms it means everything that happens around us generates invisible changes in energy fields that are detected energetically by the body's intelligence and 'transduced' into a reciprocal energy-in-motion or 'e-motion' as shown in *Figure 1*. My belief is that part of the process involves the unconscious use of our Limbic System. This system is otherwise known as the emotional brain and must be involved in 'transduction' of the energy into 'e-motion'. How exactly this happens I am not sure but I would imagine information received from the optic nerves and other senses, perhaps even the six sense, is fed to this collection of neural tissue and through a series of neurochemical signals it creates the energy-in-motion within the cells of our body. We will revisit this when we look at the effect of 'e-motions'. What we do know is this process happens before any conscious or 'head' activity can be detected even with sophisticated brain activity studies, which again points towards our claim that the 'body' is the boss and source of 'e-motion' long before the 'head' gets involved.

Let's look at a common everyday example of an 'e-motion'

being created and this should not be difficult considering we are sent a constant stream of them every day.

It is 9.30am on a Monday morning and George has had a bad weekend with burst pipes, angry wife and screaming kids. He arrives to work late for his 9.15am meeting aware that his body is sending him residual angry 'e-motion' from his disastrous weekend. Unfortunately his boss is not pleased nor willing to let it go so the lecture begins. The words, tone of voice, look on his boss's face and the sense of smugness from the boss's pet employee; all generate a negative energy in the room. If we were able to, we may see this as a dirty, red vibration that surrounded George and approached his body. The body intelligence detects this and through 'transduction' of this energy converts it into the 'energies-in-motion' of frustration and anger that arise within the cells of his body. All this happens so quickly that his head has not had the chance to pass judgement. So it begins as a protective 'e-motion' (energy-in-motion) that body intelligence sends through his cells to warn him that he is being unfairly treated. Then things really heat up as his head starts to magnify the significance of it and starts to think about his weekend, the smug guy, the boss's tone and soon the anger becomes barely containable. It is important to note here that the first step was the body intelligence's simple, truthful 'transduction' of the energy starting to surround him into an 'energy-in-motion' or 'e-motion'.

Before we look at the effects of these 'energies-in-motions' on cellular function we need to summarise some points:

- **'E-motions' are the body intelligence's energetic assessment of the world around us.**
- **They are protective though sometimes painful.**
- **They are truthful and a reflection of who we are.**
- **They are fact.**

- **They seek action to resolve situations that we face.**
- **They can be felt within our physical bodies and are therefore changing cellular function.**

Let us now look in the next chapter how they alter how our cells function.

Chapter 4

A Theory of Vibration

In order to understand this theory, we apply what we have discussed to this point concerning the fact that everything is just energy vibrating at different frequencies. The desk I am sitting at is made of wood but if we break this down further from a quantum physicist's point of view it is made of the same base building block as my hand that rests upon it. The difference is, my hand has the vibrational energy of life energy (or my spirit) within it.

My cells are therefore governed by this frequency of vibration of 'life energy'. This in turn dictates how they function. Let us use the simplistic diagram below to start to understand what I mean by this.

Figure 2

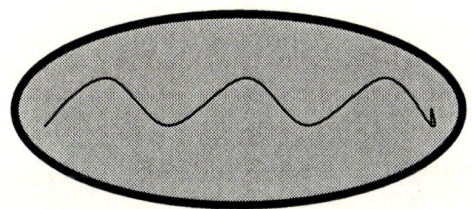

Figure 2 represents the hypothetical healthy vibrational frequency (shown as wave form) of any cell in the human body when it is functioning properly - that is in health. In other words the cell's mitochondria (otherwise known as the cell's powerhouses) are metabolising fuel compounds such as glucose, fat and proteins at an appropriate rate; the DNA is uncoiling and forming new cells at intended rates; protein production for chemicals such as hormones and other cellular products is optimal.

This is the ideal state for the human organism to exist in homeostatic health. However looking at what happens when the body intelligence creates an 'energy-in-motion', as described in the previous chapter, gives a very different picture indeed as we see in *Figure 2* below.

Figure 2

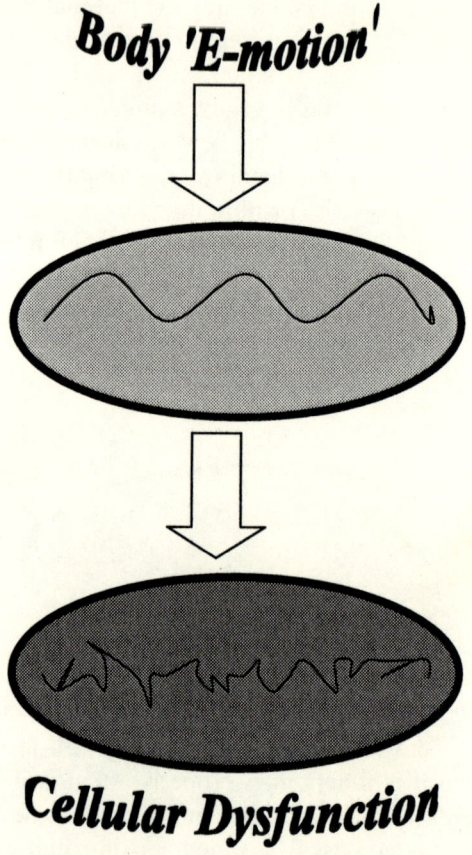

As we see above the body intelligently 'transduces' the energy of the situation into an 'e-motion' that arises within the cells and disturbs the optimal vibrational frequency of its function. This is of course is the hypothetical effect of a 'negative e-motion' it is entirely conceivable on the other hand that when the body-mind sends a positive one that cell function is enhanced.

As the negative 'e-motion' spreads through the cells, function is disturbed as the vibration is altered. This would cause numerous effects on the cells ability to do all the things it is asked to as desicribed above. Namely its metabolism, self-reproduction, protein production and general stability would be detrimentally affected. I personally think that, although diet, smoking and other factors play a role, this is the most important factor in the development of 'dis-ease'. Literally this means that the cells and therefore the organs and glands are going to cease to be at 'ease' and our most common disorders will occur such as cancer, heart disease, arthritis and many other chronic illness. This may go some way to explaining the discrepancy in prevalence of such diseases. For example, it is a well-known medical statistic that lung cancer is more prevalent in the United Kingdom than say in Spain where smoking is heavier and a more common habit. Medical research struggles to explain this. I would suggest this is a direct effect of environmental energy, how it is transduced into 'e-motions' and the difference in the cultural handling of this 'energy-in-motion' that differs between the two countries.

Similarly scientist have studied Indian tribes in the Amazon who are not only heavy smokers but also consume large quantities of home distilled alcohol of incredible volume. Now, this does not sound so different from the culture I was brought up in, but the amazing observation that has been made in these people is, as they get older they appear to get fitter and have more physical strength. As their villages can be several tens of miles apart they rely on messenger runners to go between each of them. Amazingly the best runners are the elders of the tribes and it is these villagers who are tasked with running phenomenal distances between the villages everyday. Observations suggest that these people get more capable of this the older they get! Maybe there is hope for us all yet?

To illustrate further the effect of different energies and 'e-motions' on cells; some very interesting work has been done by Dr Masaru Emoto of the I.H.M. General Research Institute in his book "Messages from Water." Dr Emoto and his colleagues discovered some startling things when they started to look at different frozen water crystals under high-powered photographic microscopes. Firstly they took water samples from different cities and nature throughout the world. Even these were spectacular in their different forms: tap water from central London and Japan (both deemed as 'stressful' cities) when viewed under microscopy showed very disturbed and poor crystal formation: water from peaceful country lakes showed beautiful stable crystal formation. Now, water is water so the clear difference between these two samples is the energy of the environment they 'inhabit'. Even more astonishing were their findings of the effect on the control water samples exposed to music, human 'e-motions' and incredibly the written word. The same sample of water would respond entirely differently to say Chopin as compared to heavy metal music - in the Chopin group the water crystals formed beautiful complexes of vibrant shapes and colours, while in the heavy metal music they became dull, distorted and lacking in structure. Similarly when the same water was exposed to 'e-motions' such as peace, calm and compassion they settled into the most magnificent shapes and literally looked 'happy' under the microscope. In contrast when exposed to 'e-motions' such as anger and hatred they became dull, distorted and formless. Perhaps even more astonishing is the effect of the water being left to sit on a piece of paper with the words 'anger' / 'hate' or 'beautiful' / 'thank you' that showed similar disturbance or enhancement respectively. When we consider that the human body is made up principally of water then we may be better able to understand the effect of 'emotions' upon our cells as described above.

Hopefully we are now getting a clearer picture of the

importance of the role of body intelligence in constantly assessing the energetic meaning of our environment and sending us **necessary** and **useful** messages about it. However this is just the beginning. In order to protect us fully it must store our experiences for future reference. It does this in the form of memory at cell level.

Chapter 5

Cellular Memory

As the body intelligence continues to assess our world and its experiences of it while creating 'energies-in-motion', its job would not be complete if it did not remember these for future reference. Otherwise we would continue to be exposed to situations that contained energy of a detrimental nature - this would be highly unsatisfactory.

Fortunately our body has the ability to store the 'energies-in-motion' at a cellular level. Therefore this becomes body memory or what has been referred to as State Dependant Memory. In Ernest Rossi's work "The Psychobiology of Mind-Body Healing" he describes this phenomenon in incredible detail both physiologically and intellectually. Here, however, I would like to give a simple overview of this important and useful phenomenon.

Firstly it is important to realise we are describing the body's intelligent memory and not that of our 'head-mind'. This is subtly different since that of the body is at an unconscious cell level. When the body deems it necessary to recall this memory, we will feel it physically as a sensation of 'e-motion' as it alters cell function.

The reader is asked to remember the series of events portrayed in *Figure 2* in the previous chapter: whereby the body intelligence transduces the energy of any given situation into 'energy-in-motion' which in turn alters the frequency of cellular vibration and its energetic content. Assuming that the situation generating this effect is resolved (to the body's satisfaction) then the transduction ceases and the cell should return to its normal frequency of vibration. Following this, the body's intelligence creates a blueprint of this 'energy-in-motion' within the cells chemically and stores it for future reference. In this way the body is able to continue to keep us protected in an unpredictable world by storing energetic experiences to serve as warning signals at a future time. These can then be released chemically and energetically from our cells as 'e-motions' and the physical sensation (symptom) of them.

Looking at some examples shows us the importance of this act of body intelligence:

- *A client of mine once came to see me with acute anxiety states that had started for the first time. Taking a history from her revealed she had never before experienced these symptoms and she was now 32 years old. The only point of interest was she had recently got a job working in an Abbey's shop that sold bits and bobs including natural wax candles. She described her work as wonderful, nice people, good hours and her home life was unchanged and happy. As I remembered what I was starting to accept in my work, namely, that all symptoms were helpful and necessary communication from the body to protect us I began to ask if she had experienced anything in her life before that her body may have been unhappy about similar to now. She could think of nothing. As I sat feeling a bit despondent that there was nothing obvious to work with, I had an idea it may well be fruitful to ask her mother if anything untoward had happened when she was very young. My reasons for doing this were that I know that body memory is always longer than the 'head's. Mary agreed to speak to her parents before her next appointment.*
When she returned next time she excitedly told me that her mum thought she might have a clue. When Mary was 18 months old it was her elder sister's seventh birthday and her mum had baked a beautiful cake that had taken all day while her sister was at school. In the evening they sat around

*the table and waited for the sister to blow out the glowing **candles**. At 18 months old Mary was very excited and couldn't get close enough to the cake and these glowing things. Unfortunately in her attempts to do so she pulled the tablecloth off and the cake followed in quick pursuit to its messy demise upon the floor. Now, although Mary's mum tried to hide her anger at all her hard work going to ruin, she did remember having to spend about an hour convincing Mary it was not the end of the world and that she was sorry she had shouted at her. This was a clue indeed and gives the perfect example of Mary's body intelligence doing its work by creating a cellular 'energy-in-motion' memory of this. Questioning Mary further it became obvious she had never realised it before, but she never had any candles for birthdays or for any other occasion for that matter and had never really given it a second thought until now. So as Mary started her new job surrounded by beautiful lit candles the body memory kicked in for the first time in 29 years to remind her of the situation that had resulted in her being shouted at and the shame she had felt. This body cellular memory was necessary and useful despite being very uncomfortable for her. The course of her treatment involved me working with her to create a new body chemical memory relating to candles. This was really quite easy and involved desensitisation techniques I had been taught in my training. Her anxiety was no longer necessary, as the new state dependant memory was that candles were indeed safe if handled properly. Mary still works in the shop and I really appreciate my annual gift of honeycombed bees wax candles.*

♦ *My wife has always called me 'Davidopoulo' due*

*to the fact that she is Greek. Then one day she decides that she has reason to be angry with me about something (of which I am sure I was innocent, by the way). During the verbal roasting I received and while ducking plates as they spun across the room at me, I noticed that suddenly I was being called 'David'. My body intelligence absorbed and transduced the energy of this situation into several 'energies-in-motion' and stored them at cell level. Now anytime she refers to me as 'David' my body triggers the release of these chemical memories and I am then warned of the trouble that could lie ahead. I then have time to decide what to do. I find running is best. My body intelligence has never been wrong yet – but I would not expect it to be – it is after all the '**Boss**'. (But please don't tell my wife this!).*

In both the cases above the body 'e-motion' was a chemical memory of fear. When the body triggered the recall of this state, several cellular changes occurred spontaneously in different tissues of the body. This included an increased adrenal cell production of the proteins used to build adrenaline, corticoids and catecholamines that then flooded our blood streams. These chemicals are associated with 'fight or flight' phenomenon and caused amongst other things increased heart rate, diversion of blood from our core to our muscles so that they would have the fuel necessary to 'get us out of there', dilatation of our pupils to allow more information (about flying plates) to be picked up. These changes in turn have an effect on our muscle tone, speed of reflexes, bowel contraction (peristalsis) and many other bodily functions.

I hope from the above examples you can start to appreciate the chemical, state dependant memories that the body creates. Please realise that neither Mary nor myself would say these cellular memories being triggered was either comfortable or enjoyable. These points are most important to understand about state dependant memories they are:

- *Often uncomfortable unless their energetic content is of a positive 'e-motion'.*
- *Frequent and never run out until no longer necessary (as with Mary)*
- ***Helpful and necessary communication from our body.***

In other words we should be thankful for them.

Chapter 6

So what are 'Symptoms'?

Symptoms are traditionally associated with illness. They are therefore the subjective experience of any condition of 'dis-ease'. This means they are unwanted, troublesome sensations that arise in our physical bodies. However I hope through reading this short book that the reader is already starting to get a different perspective on them.

They are undoubtedly experienced as uncomfortable, and so they should, because they are the body's intelligent way of communicating some 'dis-ease' that it is experiencing. Throughout my medical training I was taught to approach them as things to get rid of. Unfortunately I realise now that this was achieved, more often than not, by finding ways to put them to sleep or in other words 'shoot the messenger'. This is a pity since I know now the message of the symptom is actually **useful** and **necessary.** This should sound familiar to the reader since we have used this term throughout to describe 'e-motions' and the state dependant chemical memory of them.

Symptoms are therefore the physical sensation of the 'energy-in-motion' whether it be acutely transduced from the environment or re-released from state dependant memory. In other words as a continuation of *Figure 2:*

Figure 3

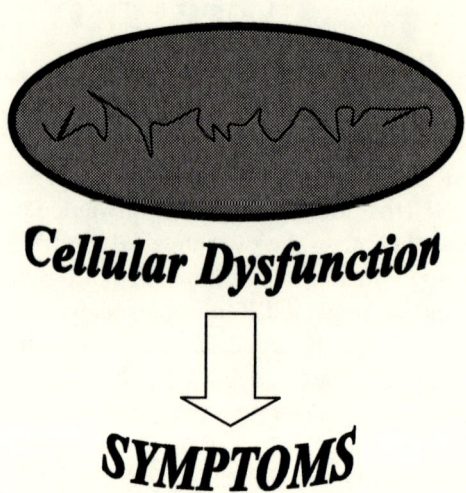

Cellular Dysfunction

⇩

SYMPTOMS

**Metabolic change
Hormone production altered
Neurochemical output level
Cell Reproduction rate
(Blood supply altered)**

In *Figure 3* we start to see how firstly, the cell dysfunction takes place that spreads throughout the relevant tissue disturbing many of its functions. These then create the physical symptoms. It is important to keep in mind however that by retracing the arrows (from *Figures 3 back to 1)* we always come back to the original source of all this - namely the energetic transduction of the energy of the environmental situation into 'energy-in-motion' by the body intelligence in an effort to communicate to us its evaluations of our world in general.

An example of this from my own experiences would be through the very common symptoms of IBS or Irritable Bowel Syndrome. When I was working in General Practice my IBS was at its worst. The situational energy my body transduced into 'e-motion' was related to the bizarre fashion in which the Government set up of the NHS, long working hours, too much pointless paperwork to have any time for patients and the local politics or lack of them within my Practice. The label I would now give to this 'energy-in-motion' would be 'frustration'. This energy then at a cellular level disrupted the normal function of my bowel and its subsequent reaction to food, thus creating bloating, pain, gas and frequent visits to the toilet. Interestingly, as I approached this more from a Mickel Therapy perspective and started to deal with the request of this communication from my body intelligence, my symptoms lessened until by the time I left General Practice I had almost no symptoms and was able to eat most of the things that previously had not been tolerated. The food intolerances were an **effect** of the 'energy-in-motion' on my bowel's cells and **not** the cause. I now see that had my body not done its job again and sent me symptoms as communication then I would have remained in the situation's negative energy and not started to deal with it differently. This in turn would have led to further chronic cellular disruption in my bowel (due to persistent production of 'energy-in-motion') and who knows what the effects of this would have been on my bowel's cells after 20 years. Of course because of the state dependant memory of this within my cells, I am now alerted very early to situations that are creating the 'e-motion' of frustration - this gives me the chance to respond differently to things and avoid future chronic frustration for which I thank my body wholeheartedly.

Where purely 'physiological' symptoms fit in

Such symptoms as hunger, thirst and healthy tiredness are

obviously not generated through the transduction of **external** situational energy. They are however results of the transduction of **internal** changes in energy. For example if my blood glucose drops this results in a specific change in the energy that it provides to maintain the vibartional frequency of my cells. My body intelligence then creates the symptom of hunger associated with a need for sugar. If I respond to this appropriately by eating enough of this then the energy change returns to normal and my body stops sending the symptom as a messenger to communicate with me.

So in summary symptoms are:

- **Created at cell level by 'energies-in-motion' and the effect of these on cell function by altering the vibrational frequency.**
- **Helpful and necessary communication from the body although often experienced as uncomfortable.**
- **Contained within the cells as state dependant chemical memory.**
- **Always protective.**
- **To be listened to and responded to appropriately so that they can stop being produced.**
- **NOT to be 'shot down' with medication.**

Now that we have a basic understanding of body intelligence, 'energies-in-motion', cellular memory, and the necessity of symptoms we can now go on to look at the conditions of Chronic Fatigue Syndrome, ME and Fibromyalgia or as Mickel Therapy calls it **'Hypothalamitis'**.

Chapter 7

Chronic Fatigue Syndrome, ME and Fibromyalgia

Since so much has already been written about the conditions to little avail, I would like to just summarise some of the details in the following. I hope it will be useful at some practical level.

These conditions are now reaching epidemic proportions worldwide - especially in the Western world. Some sources believe that the prevalence could be as high as 1% in any given population. This is a shocking fact and it is a wonder that more progress has not been made in treating them. Or perhaps it is not. One of the most frustrating aspects of the conditions for a medical practitioner is not just having nothing to offer as treatment, but also the lack of hard tests to arrive at the diagnosis in the first place.

Mickel Therapy views the conditions as all part of the same spectrum of disease, namely 'Hypothalamitis'. I am aware this causes some disagreement amongst sufferers but I am confident that it is the case. If it were not the case then our treatment would not have equal success in all three disorders.

Diagnosis

It is likely that there are several thousand sufferers more in the United Kingdom alone who have these conditions but have not been given a diagnosis. These individuals are likely to have a lower severity of symptoms and therefore continue to plod on through life with less energy and enjoyment. Indeed, we have seen more and more cases of this nature recently but fortunately their recovery rate can be very rapid following Mickel Therapy.

In 2002 after four years 'study' the CMO for England and Wales published the results of his Working Group Report.

This made disappointing reading for sufferers especially when the suggested treatment involved Cognitive Behavioural Therapy - that as we already know, doesn't offer a cure - although it may help sufferers to cope better with their illness. Of course it is no surprise it doesn't work considering that it has already been shown to be ineffective. It is however slightly surprising that the Working Group took 4 years to come up with this suggested treatment considering that has already shown to be ineffective!

However some useful information came out of the Report surrounding guidance for diagnosing cases by Doctors. The purpose of the steps involved is to establish a **diagnosis of exclusion.** This means quite simply that all other conditions have to be ruled out before a Doctor considers giving a diagnosis. Fortunately this is not difficult to do and the tests are simple to take. The following is taken from the Working Group Report 2002 and details the test that Doctors are advised to do when presented with a case of someone with a six months history of significant fatigue with pain in their muscles and joints and other symptoms such as sore throats, enlarged glands, intolerances to food, headaches etc.

Tests

Full Clinical History and Physical examination
Mental Health evaluation - to exclude depressive illness (please see later chapter)
Assessment of sleep - to exclude pre-existing primary sleep disturbance
Basic Blood test -
- *Full blood count* - this looks for anaemia and signs of immune system problems.
- *CRP* - this is reactive protein and is a general indicator of inflammation or disease process in the body.

- *Blood Biochemistry* - this looks at kidney function, liver function, blood glucose, thyroid function.

Specimen of urine - not quite sure why we do these since anything detected here would also have shown up in the above tests. I suppose it could exclude urinary infection and double check for blood loss and diabetes.

Specialist tests - only indicated if the above suggest the possibility of other disorders that may need referral to specialist.

If the above criteria are met and the tests do not reveal any other disorder then the diagnosis of exclusion is arrived at.

Chapter 8

The Condition of 'Hypothalamitis'

Before looking at the state of 'Hypothalamitis' an understanding of the Hypothalamus in health is necessary.

Very little mention of the Hypothalamus was made during my medical studies. More often, if mentioned, it was in conjunction with the Pituitary gland and the Hypothalamic-Pituitary-Adrenal axis. Indeed, this is the pathway between the Hypothalamus, Pituitary and the Adrenal glands that has been the focus of much research into the conditions of CFS/ME and Fibromyalgia. However this is only a small part of the involvement of the Hypothalamus in maintaining a healthy physiological environment within the human body.

Conventionally the Pituitary has been viewed as the 'Master Gland', but this has to be inaccurate since its functions are in turn governed by the Hypothalamus. As we will see, the Hypothalamus is the **true** 'Master Gland' and is directly or indirectly involved in every function of the human body. Therefore, it is little wonder that should it start to dysfunction ('Hypothalamitis') then the effects of this on our body's function would be significant.

In health the Hypothalamus is responsible for homeostasis - that is to keep everything in a balanced equilibrium of health. It does this by being involved in an intricate feedback mechanism whereby physiological changes within the whole body are relayed back to the Hypothalamus and it makes the necessary alterations in hormone secretion and neural signals to counteract these effects. In this way it is like a central processor, constantly receiving information and making informed decisions as to what needs to be done about it.

Incredibly the Hypothalamus gland is barely pea-sized in the adult human and yet its role is unarguably the most important.

In the state of 'Hypothalamitis', which literally means an inflamed Hypothalamus, we hypothesise that its signals to the body go into overdrive. The effect of this is basically to overdrive our systems and not respond to their requests (through the feedback mechanism) for rest - thus resulting in a never-ending state of extreme overwork with all the symptoms associated with this.

The Symptoms of 'Hypothalamitis'

The symptoms involved in the conditions of CFS, ME and Fibromyalgia are part of a wide spectrum of suffering. I will discuss the most predominant ones below in relation to this causal state of 'Hypothalamitis' with the aid of *Figure 4* that is adapted from the work of Hans Selye from the 1930's.

Figure 4

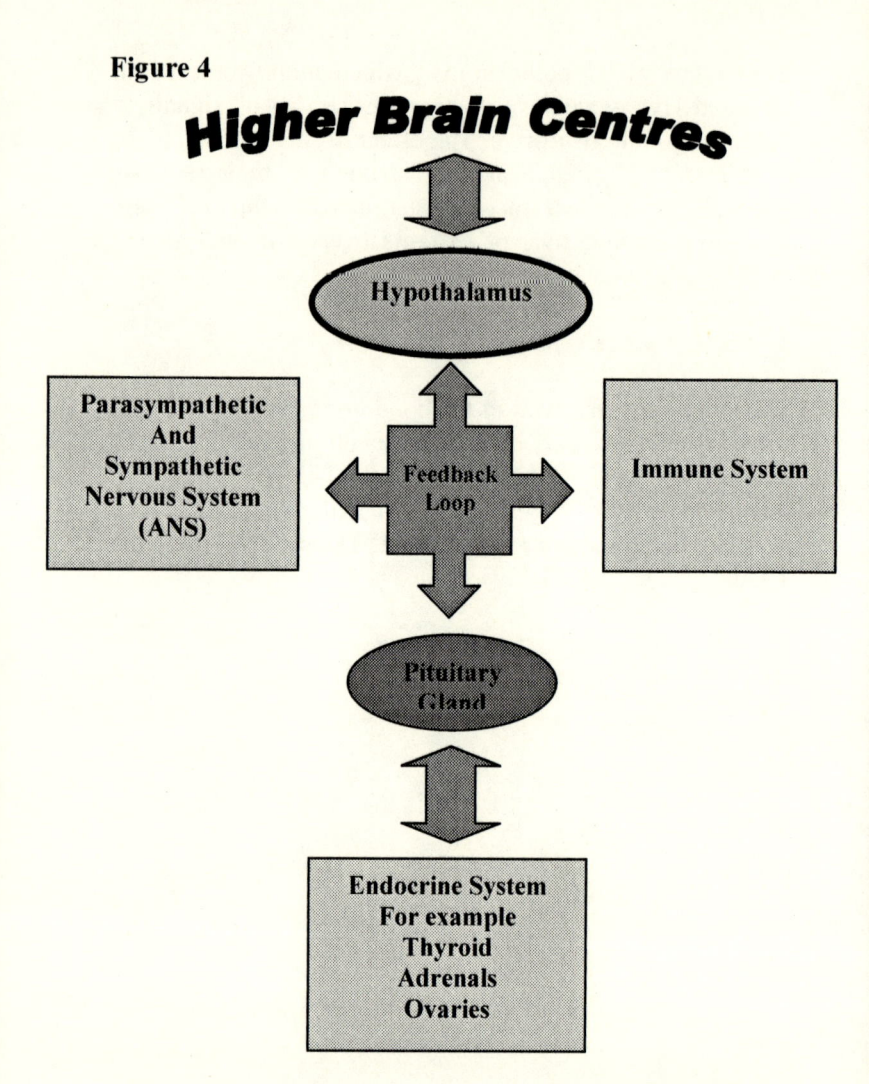

Higher Brain Centres

```
           Hypothalamus
                ↕
Parasympathetic
And
Sympathetic    ← Feedback →   Immune System
Nervous System    Loop
(ANS)
                ↕
           Pituitary
           Gland
                ↕
        Endocrine System
         For example
           Thyroid
           Adrenals
           Ovaries
```

Figure 4 – Is a simplified diagrammatic representation of the Hypothalamus and its connections within the human. Please note that, as represented by the central arrow, everything is interconnected and therefore communicating with neuro-chemical signals. In this way we can see how changes in one area will have an affect throughout all our systems. Of most importance, is to see how the Hypothalamus has the pivotal governing role over all functions. Bearing this in mind let us now look at the explanation of some of the major symptoms of 'Hypothalamitis' - otherwise referred to as CFS, ME and Fibromyalgia.

- ♦ **Fatigue** - this is a very subjective experience but well known to all of us. However the fatigue generated in 'Hypothalamitis' is staggering and unless suffered can only be compared by the rest of us to our state dependant memories of our worse lethargy following a very bad flu. Interestingly the effect of the release of the toxins from viruses, especially influenza, is to stimulate an acute effect on the Hypothalamus akin to 'Hypothalamitis'. Although this fatigue is a mixture of very complicated chemical and cellular change, simplistically it can be explained by the following.

  The state of 'Hypothalamitis', through the pituitary gland, stimulates the release of a large array of chemicals from the Adrenal Glands including adrenaline, catecholamines and corticoids. These can be referred to as 'chemicals of exertion' that are carried in our blood throughout our body. Although they have many effects on our cells, the predominant one, in my opinion is on the muscle cells where they cause a chemically induced state of exertion. That is to say, they increase muscle cell metabolism, increase isotonic tone and effectively make the muscles work very hard - even when we are at rest. This explains the phenomenon in the conditions of CFS, ME and Fibromyalgia whereby sufferers describe going to bed for 12 hours or more and when they awake their muscles feel like they have been running a marathon. In chemical terms this is exactly what they have been doing while the person 'rested'. Since the muscles require energy to do this they then deplete the body's energy stores and this leads to further fatigue as the mitochondria work overtime. This explains what researchers are noting in studying muscle metabolism and levels of cyclical AMP, ATP etc. However, these are **effects** and not the **cause** of the conditions and further research will be fruitless. In normal Hypothalamus function the feedback loop would warn the Hypothalamus that the body and especially muscles were overworking and it would alter its signals through the Pituitary and Adrenals and reduce the production of these chemicals of 'exertion'. Unfortunately in 'Hypothalamitis' it appears to respond by further increasing demand in this way and the individual enters into a vicious circle of never ending chemical exertion and fatigue. It is then little wonder that further attempts to use the muscles for actual movement results in overwhelming fatigue.

- **Myalgia (muscle pain)** - this is easily explained by the above phenomenon. Muscles that work, whether chemical or actual, produce by-products of this exertion through metabolism. The main by-product is lactic acid. This is generated when the glucose is used without enough oxygen for its full metabolism i.e anaerobic. Lactic acid is the chemical that gives the effect that we have all experienced the day or so after hard physical exercise. In fact, as I write this book I am aware of a build up of this in my hand and forearm muscles following days on end of typing. I know that this will clear when I stop this exertion, while in the conditions I describe ('Hypothalamitis') this does not happen because the muscles are continually exerted chemically. This explains the painful muscles and trigger points described especially in Fibromyalgia.

- **Arthralgia (joint pain)** - since there has not been found, despite numerous studies, any convincing evidence of joint pathology in these conditions then how come this symptom is experienced by so many? My opinion is, the most likely explanation is that it is actually referred pain. This means it does not arise in the joints but rather in areas around the joints that have the same nervous supply. This is a common phenomenon in medicine and there are many examples of it such as when we have trapped nerve in our neck (the accessory nerve) we then experience the pain between our shoulder blades. Or equally in the case of sciatica, the pain is felt down the back of the leg and into the foot, instead of in our backs where the trouble lies. So, in this way, remembering the tone is increased subtly in these chemically exerting muscles, slight strain is placed upon the areas where the muscles attach around the joint and this may create some inflammation over time, which is detected by the same nerves that serve the joints themselves and is therefore experienced as joint pain.

- **Headache** - this common symptom occurs in cases to different degrees and seems to be most predominant in the early stages of 'Hypothalamitis'. Its cause is multifactorial including effects of adjusting to visual disturbance and lack of restful sleep. However I think the most likely cause of this troublesome symptom is explained by the theory explained above of chronic, intractable muscle exertion. Since the human scalp is muscular and it too is therefore increasing in tone and subtly shrinking around the fixed mass of the skull, then it makes sense that this would explain the subjective experience of band like headaches and pain above the eyes and back of the neck where the muscles attach.

- **Visual disturbance** - again there are wide variety of forms of this described by sufferers of 'Hypothalamitis'. Principally they are caused by the chemical muscular exertion effect on the eye muscles used for movement that make even the slightest eye movement a painful chore, the effect of inappropriate stimulation of the pupil muscle by the ANS (autonomic nervous system) resulting in light sensitivity and the effect on the muscles that alter the shape of the lenses to focus that results in blurring of vision.

- **Vertigo and balance disturbance** - many different effects of 'Hypothalamitis' combine to create these effects. These include: the stimulation of the ANS (through the lateral medulla) and adrenaline to divert blood to the muscles that takes it away from our brains, resulting in an effective drop in blood pressure which manifests as dizziness especially on bending down or standing up too quickly - otherwise known as ' orthostatic hypotension'; stimulation of the immune system (see below) to act as if infection was present that leads to an increase in mucous within the middle ear and disturbs the effectiveness of our balance control where it is situated in the form of the Vestibulo-Cochlear cells.

- **Concentration and memory impairment** - to attempt to fully understand this phenomenon would take more knowledge than I possess of neuropsychophysiology. However we do have some clues. Most people with 'Hypothalamitis' suffer from a degree of sleep disturbance (see below) and we know that sleep is essential for processing and storing memory as well as making us more able to concentrate. It makes sense that these two abilities are going to be reduced following sleep disturbance. Also human thought starts in the frontal lobe and spreads like a chemical and electrical wave across the hemispheres of our brain to be processed into memory and understanding in the posterior lobe. I envisage this is a little like a radio wave in form and as it passes over the brain it encounters interference from the waves being produced by the overactive 'Hypothalamitis'. This must surely cause some interference of our thought waves and render them less than clear by the time that they reach the posterior lobe.

- **Insomnia and hypersomnia** - in other words lack of or too much sleep respectfully. Sleep is governed by a natural biorhythm that alters between phases of rest and arousal at 40-90 minute intervals. In 'Hypothalamitis' the time between each phase is shortened due to the general speeding up of every system as it responds to the Hypothalamus. This has two effects depending on the relative increase in rate. In insomnia people describe just getting off to sleep and then waking up soon after as they experience the return of the arousal phase - all too soon. This is clearly not conducive to restful sleep and the necessary alpha and delta brainwaves are not reached in time. Occasionally, especially early in the condition of 'Hypothalamitis', hypersomnia occurs. That is the individual sleeps constantly for hours and hours per day and night without feeling regenerated. During this, usually acute spell, I would say the biorhythm is speeded up to such a rate that the troughs of the rest phases merge to form one prolonged rest phase of endless sleepiness.

♦ **Altered resistance to common infections** – this phenomenon is the result of the state of 'Hypothalamitis' on the immune system. Initially there is probably an increase in Immune system cell production in response to the Hypothalamus's demand for work. This results in an acute stage of optimum cell-mediated immunity. This is short lived and soon the cellular immunity cannot maintain this and it crashes lower than normal levels. It is at this time that opportunistic infections enter our body, such as Epstein Barr, influenza, coxsackie A & B etc. This is the reason why I do not believe that infections cause the conditions of CFS, ME or Fibromyalgia. When looking closely at cases there is evidence of the 'Hypothalamitis' condition subtly sending symptoms prior to the infection. Infections are therefore an effect of an existing 'Hypothalamitis' case developing and **not** cause of it. This means the diagnosis of Post Viral Fatigue Syndrome is meaningless and misleading.

Following this initial rise and then crash of the immune system, one of two things happens that will decide whether the sufferer of 'Hypothalamitis' gets recurrent infections or more fortunately almost none. I have seen this distinct division of clients over the last 4 years and from my records it looks like 65% of sufferers have a super immune system. They describe almost no upper respiratory tract infections despite all around them decimating rain forests with their use of

Kleenex. This can only be explained by the fact that after crashing, their immune system, under constant stimulation by the effect of the 'Hypothalamitis' manages to pick itself up and rise above normal levels of immunity with increased defence against infections. The other 35% however report recurrent viral infections and their immune system obviously did not recover from the initial crash. The good news is that in all the cases Mickel Therapy has treated both these groups seem to return to normal levels. Unfortunately this does mean that the group of super immune systems may get occasional colds etc but most would agree this is a small price to pay.

♦ **Temperature changes** - clients describe varying signs of temperature fluctuations from heat to suddenly cold. This is explained by the fact that the Thermoregulatory centre is centred within the Hypothalamus gland itself. Between about 18 months old and 3 years this is in a rapid stage of development and is extremely sensitive to effects of viral exotoxins. This explains the prevalence of febrile convulsions in children of this age. In 'Hypothalamitis' the cellular disruption of the gland means it ceases to effectively control core temperature and this results in it trying to increase it or decrease it randomly. This leads to the subjective experience of being too hot or too cold as the skin blood flow is altered to either conserve heat energy or radiate more of it respectively.

♦ **Chronic signs of a 'head cold'** - symptoms of this include blocked sinuses, enlarged glands (especially in the neck), red and sore throats and sore or blocked ears. In my work in General Practice I came across these symptoms and signs regularly in sufferers of 'Hypothalamitis' and I tried to find evidence of infection from viral blood tests, throat and nasopharyngeal swabs. In almost all cases these tests were negative. I then realised that although these symptoms and signs suggested infection there was not in fact one present. I think this is caused by the 'Hypothalamitis' creating an immune cellular state dependent memory. In other words these areas were acting as if they remembered an infection by increasing mucous production in the sinuses and ears (often causing pain or sensitivity to sound), increased lymphatic fluid in the glands that made them swell and blood was diverted to the pharynx (throat) to bring immune cells to the first line of attack. In this way the body was being made ready for viral attack just in case.

♦ **Indigestion, nausea, bloating, diarrhoea, and apparent food intolerances** - these are commonly described by those with 'Hypothalamitis'. My impression is that these are caused by a combination of over stimulated ANS (Autonomic Nervous System), especially the Vagus nerve causing increased stomach acidity, reduced stomach emptying by tightening the pyloric valve which allows contents out of the stomach, and increasing peristalsis - the contractions of the bowel - leading to diarrhoea (although constipation is occasionally mentioned). This combined with an over sensitive immune cell response to previously innocuous, food compounds creates the development of intolerances to them. Over a period of time, the increased stomach acidity and the subsequent bowel attempts to alkalise this effect, recurrent antibiotics and prolonged diarrhoea the healthy flora in the bowel diminishes and creates a very habitable growing environment for *candida albicans*. Again it is important to realise that the candida infection is an effect of the 'Hypothalamitis' and **not** a cause. Dietary attempts to deal with this are both restrictive and only palliative since the only way to return things to normal is to treat the cause - 'Hypothalamitis'. I have treated many cases with this complication and never had to alter diets. Once the 'Hypothalamitis' is put back to normal and the effect described above is reversed then the candida soon departs.

Chapter 9

This is not Depression!

I can't tell you how many times I have met clients who have had the suggestion made to them that they may have depression and have either been sent to a local Psychiatrist or started on medication. In 90% of cases this is simply not true. If it is true then they have it as a separate condition. Having said that I have to admit, in my early exposure to CFS, ME and Fibromyalgia it did seem a reasonable suggestion. I soon realised, however, that the conditions were not the same at all. Let us remind ourselves that CFS, ME and Fibromyalgia are a physical condition caused by a dysfunction of the Hypothalamus gland that we call 'Hypothalamitis'. They are **not** examples of depression. This again explains the folly of trying to treat people with psychological treatments.

Of course this does not mean to say that after years of suffering people will not get lowering of their affect and mood to different degrees - this would be classified as a form of depression. But again this is an effect **not** a cause. In these cases, the brain serotonin levels undoubtedly drop and this explains the partial improvement felt by people who have taken the usual antidepressants. However this does not treat the 'Hypothalamitis' and the symptoms do not stop. The only way to treat this secondary depression is to remove the cause - namely by treating the 'Hypothalamitis'.

People can get the conditions of 'Hypothalamitis' and depression co-existently. Therefore all Mickel Therapists are trained to treat the condition of depression as well.

Chapter 10

Mickel Therapy Treatment - what to expect.

I will describe in some brief detail the process that the client will experience if they do decide to receive our treatment. Remember this is a talking therapy - nothing else. The sessions take place face to face just between therapist and client. Third parties are not invited into the session primarily because, when I used to allow this to happen, I found that the treatments took much longer to reach cure - I think this was because it led to 'head' discussions outside the room. It is for this reason we ask clients not to discuss treatment until they are completely better and then they can talk about it until their hearts are content.

Hopefully before starting treatment you will have read this book thoroughly and understood its principals. I am confident this will shorten your treatment and make it easier.

We will now look at an overview of the sessions that tend to be about an hour long. Remember that Mickel Therapy has been designed to treat people who are both extremely fatigued and find concentrating and memorising difficult, the process takes this into account.

Sessions 1-2 - these sessions are primarily for getting a history from the client, answering their questions, explaining the symptoms in terms of 'Hypothalamitis' to check that this is accepted. Usually in the second session (although this may be later in some cases) the therapist will then work with you to explore the symptoms in terms of body intelligent communication. The therapist is trained to interpret and then translate the literal message that the body wants to be received when it sends symptoms as a state dependent memory. This is what we call 'easing out the message'.

Sessions 3 onwards - client and therapist review the symptom experiences the client has had between sessions to understand more about the purpose of the symptoms and what the body intelligence needs done to be allowed to stop generating them. Every case is different, but in all of them at some point it as if the penny finally drops and the symptoms reduce and then stop coming altogether. Your therapist will then ask you to contact them after 4-6 weeks to ensure you are still well. It is very important to realise that, although a rare occurrence, if symptoms return you are encouraged to contact your therapist and be seen at short notice. In the cases where this has happened it took only 1 or 2 sessions to re-correct the situation back to a normal Hypothalamus and asymptomatic health.

A final word

Should you decide to start Mickel Therapy then I want you to feel assured that its therapists are highly trained and closely supervised in their art. I supervise their work myself and although I do not expect it to be necessary, if you do have any concerns about your treatment then please direct them to me personally. The contact details are in the Appendix following some testimonials by ex-clients who have led the way before you.

Chapter 11

Testimonials

"I had been ill for nearly five years, three years of which I had become pretty much housebound. It's hard to imagine now, so great is the contrast between then and now. I suppose the worst and most debilitating symptoms were total exhaustion, muscle pain, emotional instability and the resulting frustration and depression that followed. That's putting it mildly really.

Of course, like anyone else who is desperate to feel well again, I tried endless diets and various therapies, some of which did indeed relieve symptoms; but only the symptoms, not resolving the actual problem.

Mickel Therapy started to have a positive effect on me within a short space of time, and over the period of a few months I had returned to full health. I knew all that I had left to work on was rebuilding my physical stamina.

I can now honestly say I am totally and permanently better, and slightly more than that...in some way better equipped to deal with life, with an altered attitude which brings with it a certain sense of strength."

JB 2002

"My Fibromyalgia condition had been present for 19 years. I was in constant exhausting pain, tired and unable to take part in family life never mind even consider employment. I was hugely frustrated by the lack of success I had had with different treatments - diet, herbs, acupuncture, homeopathy - you name it, I had tried it. Over the last year before Mickel Therapy I had given into my Doctor's recommendation of a trial of antidepressants. Needless to say after 3 different types, I was still where I started off - symptoms galore, tired and losing my hope for any kind of future.

I thought I would try Mickel Therapy on the advice of a friend who had seen a presentation at a local help group. At my first session I was immediately heartened to learn that my condition was linked to something concrete and the mystery removed.

From the first session I was amazed to notice subtle improvements in the physical pains I had had for so long. Over the next few weeks my health began to improve with each session. I was amazed and can't find the words to describe the sense of relief I felt. The real test came towards the end of my treatment program when I had several unfortunate family crises. This would normally have magnified my symptoms 100 fold - but to my delight I continued to get stronger and stronger.

Eight months have passed now and I am completely better - in fact better than I ever remember feeling before. Mickel Therapy gave me back my life and I am very grateful."

RB 2003

"By the time I first saw my Mickel Therapist (in Feb 2002), I had almost given up the idea that anything could help me get better. I had been in bed for two years, although I had been struggling with life for many years previously, and had tried every 'miracle' cure out there. In March 2000 I had to leave University and go back home as I was too exhausted to cope, things went down hill very fast and soon I was living in a dark room, unable to take light or noise, with very little contact with the outside world. After a year

or so most of the symptoms (headaches, aches and pains, memory loss etc.) stopped but I still had terrible fatigue and managed, at most, an hour of activity spread through the day (chatting to my mum or watching television).
Starting Mickel Therapy was amazing, for the first time I met someone who completely understood the illness and was confident that he could help, I wasn't quite sure how he thought he was going to do it, but I put my trust in him, and will never forget what he has done for me.

It was hard work for a while, facing up to the illness and it's causes, I would quite often come out of the treatment room tired, yet always feeling a little better. Within a month I started to notice small changes in my condition, I managed a little more one week than I had the last.

The day I realized that things were changing was when I had a shower one morning before going to see my therapist. Usually when I had a shower I had to spend the rest of the day recovering and resting, going to see him had previously been a huge effort for me as we lived an hour away (getting out of bed and into the back seat of the car, the noise, the light etc). Yet I had managed both of these things in one day and felt okay the next day.

In a few weeks I was going to see him on my own, chatting to friends regularly, reading books, listening to music, slowly getting my life back on track.

I left home in August 2002 and moved down to London to live with my brother, catch up with my friends and get on with my life. As I said earlier I will never forget what Mickel Therapy has done for me. As well as giving me my life back it has also taught me a huge amount about how to live life to the full without putting my health at risk. Nowadays I take nothing for granted and enjoy everything about life, and I hope that never changes. Looking back, I wonder what would have happened if I hadn't found Mickel Therapy. I am pretty sure I would still be there, lying in bed with the curtains shut dreaming of what my life should be like, yet here I am living it."

AS 2002

"By the time I came across an article about Mickel Therapy in the 'Sunday Post', I had almost hit rock bottom and had been ill for six years. At my worst, I was mostly bedridden, only having the energy for trips from my bedroom to the bathroom. My husband had to bath, dry and dress me, cut up my food, help me up from chairs when I became 'stuck' and I even recall one occasion, (which I can laugh about now) where I asked him to squeeze the toothpaste tube for me. Life was virtually non-existent. And when you're in your early thirties with a job, husband and a toddler to look after, you'll try anything to muster up even the tiniest bit of energy.

From the moment my therapist met me, he was always insistent that I would get better. Always the pessimist, I had my doubts. I was disappointed at first, as after three treatments, there was no difference. But after the fourth, things started to change. Don't get me wrong - it didn't just happen. This is a treatment which you have to work at, and at times I found it difficult to respond to my body's message. But I soon started to reap the benefits. These tiny day- to-day things which we all take for granted suddenly became very exciting and pleasurable - ie, lifting the kettle, putting my own clothes on, reading my toddler a book, having a shower. With each treatment, I grew stronger and more positive. That awful ill feeling was starting to lift.

And where am I now? Eight months after I started

treatment I can now swim 40 lengths of the pool again, I can go out on a Saturday night and dance the night away and I can be a proper wife and mother. I just dread to think where I would be now if I hadn't picked up the phone that day and made an appointment. Thanks to Mickel Therapy and the dedication of my therapist, I now have a life again."

P S

"I am an avid reader of the Sunday Post and one Sunday I noticed an advert in it about an Elgin doctor having found a cure for Fibromyalgia called Mickel Therapy. I had a look at the website but felt a bit sceptical about it all. Was this another one of those alternative therapy practitioners out to make money out of people's suffering I thought? I was quite surprised to find there was neither drugs or hypnosis involved either which I thought was rather strange. I thought well "I have tried everything else - I may as well give this a go as well".

When I first saw my Mickel Therapist in June of 2003 although I had read about some of what the treatment actually involved I was still a bit unsure. However after that first session I realised he knew how I was feeling and what sort of symptoms I was suffering from. I was also delighted to hear that he believed my symptoms were real and not imagined (as had been the case when I went to my GP). I still remained a bit unsure of how he could help but decided to give him a chance. I came out of the first session feeling a sense of relief in that I had found someone who understood and could help me. I actually cried during that first session with the relief. It was very hard work and fairly traumatic facing up to the illness throughout and indeed finding out some of its causes as it meant me facing up to some baggage in my life I had been carrying about with me but I didn't want to think too deeply about. The Mickel Therapist treats both mind and the body and explained how closely connected both were and how one affects the other. After each session things slowly improved although I did have a few setbacks on occasion but continued with therapy and eventually found to my delight I was fully recovered.

Three months have now passed since I last saw the therapist. I am in the middle of a family crisis and moving home (we all know how stressful that can be) which would have exacerbated my symptoms greatly in the past but I find I can now cope with no more adverse reactions than the average person would have.

I can't really describe in words what Mickel Therapy has done to help me."

J.S. 2003

When I went to see my Mickel Therapist for the first time I had been unwell for 2 years. I was a little bit sceptical about going as I had seen no end of doctors in the past, and not one had managed to cure me of my ME. I had gone from being an outgoing, active teenager to a lethargic, uninterested invalid who did not want to move from the settee. Even the thought of going to school was a huge effort. Some days I couldn't even bring myself to do that.
Mickel Therapy completely cured me of my ME in less than half a year. Even after the first hour session people began to see a difference in me. When I got home from my first appointment, I immediately went and picked up a tennis racquet! That was the first time in months I had done any physical exercise.
Every time I came out of a session I felt in myself that I had made an improvement from when I went in. This encouraged me to make the extra effort and follow the advice in making myself better.

Thanks to Mickel Therapy I now have things back on track and can begin to enjoy my life again.

CW 2004

I developed ME 15 years ago following a post-operation infection. I was very ill at first with pains in my arms and legs, continuous fatigue, headaches, poor sleep and hypersensitivity to light, sound and smell. I was not totally bed-bound but was frequently forced to go back to bed because of pain and tiredness.

I was admitted to hospital and a diagnosis of ME was made by muscle biopsy.

There was a very slow improvement but I was totally house bound for years and we bought a wheelchair.

I had the best possible support from my family, and am very fortunate in my GP who totally believed in my condition, but like most people with ME, wondered if my friends thought the illness was taking too long to clear up and why I was still having to cancel or postpone arrangements.

Several drugs were tried but were ineffective and had to be stopped because of side effects. I tried alternative therapies, diets and Acupuncture.

Now after ten sessions of Mickel Therapy I have no muscle pains or overpowering fatigue. I am out of the house most for outings or to shops or for walks, and I now walk without a stick.

I travelled 100 miles to each session without undue fatigue, I found the sessions totally without stress, with good empathy and understanding and was very glad no drugs were involved.

I do not feel 100% well because the abdominal problems which preceded the ME by several years and which caused me to retire early from medical practice, are still present , and also because I am now 76 and cannot expect the energy

I would like especially after so many years of inactivity but I am very content with how I now feel.

A few months ago writing this article would have completely exhausted me!

RM 2004

About four years ago I became unwell with Glandular Fever. However, it was not the fever that caused me my major problems. After Glandular Fever I turned into an entirely different person. I became extremely tired constantly, my muscles ached every minute of the day and I could hardly do the daily things I used to be able to do. My friends could not understand why I physically was not able to go out and enjoy myself. This upset me and I became depressed.

I attended several meetings with GP's who referred me to two different paediatricians, and both separately believed this was a short-term phase of post-viral fatigue. I was told to carry on with everyday activities and was warned to do anything but rest. I was then referred to a physiotherapist who claimed I had ME. The physiotherapy helped regain some muscular strength for a short period of time. However it did not help the aching in my body or the way I felt after participating in various activities. I tried to carry on with my daily routine and continue to participate in school sports and events, as I did not want to miss out or for people to notice something was wrong and the tiredness would get me down. I did try to continue as normal but by the time I got home from school I was so tired I would collapse on the sofa and my muscles would ache even more. I still continued to have memory loss and I had lack of concentration at all times no matter what I was doing. I could not think straight and at that time I was sitting exams. The pressure and stress built up and I could not handle it.

I continued with this trauma for one year and eventually I discovered something I thought might be able to help me. I read an article in the local newspaper about a practice that had recently opened, offering Mickel Therapy, to help those with ME, and related illnesses. This was just what I needed. I was so excited at the fact that there was someone out there that might help me. I made my mother phone for an appointment immediately. I had previously tried everything available and I was willing to give anything a go. I just wanted to be back to my old self as soon as possible. I hated the way I felt.

I had my first session with my Mickel Therapist and during the session I felt brand new. I learnt that I did not have ME. In fact I had 'Hypothalamitis'. This means that one part of the brain (the Hypothalamus) had stopped functioning properly. Mickel Therapy altered the Hypothalamus and it started to function correctly again. At the end of the session my mother was invited into the room. My therapist asked her to look out for any change in my condition. She noted the immediate physical change. I was laughing. It was as if a veil had been lifted and my eyes sparkled like they used to. She said she could tell the improvement in my attitude, my outlook and my frame of mind. I had no aches or pains and I was the old me again. It felt as though these problems had stopped instantaneously. After one session I was cured. It was amazing. I returned for another meeting, not for treatment, but to record my progress. I did not need to return for treatment again. It was a miracle - completely surreal, but remarkable. I did not think I would be my normal self again until I discovered Mickel Therapy.

It is one year now since I have been cured from Hypothalamitis. I continue to go about my everyday business like I always used to before my illness. I still cannot believe how lucky I was to have that chance. It really has changed my life. It saved me and my mother says she now has her daughter back.

EM 2004

I was diagnosed as suffering from ME 18 years ago in the days when 'yuppie flu' hit the headlines. I was told that no coordinated treatment was available within the NHS as the cause was unknown and there was still disbelief that this was an illness. I envisaged a future of depressing hopelessness with some terrifying symptoms that defy imagination and a fatigue beyond the recognized description of the word.

From being healthy, active and energetic I felt my chemical body was completely out of control. I lived with constant pain, fatigue and frustration as to how little help was available.

Over the years a plethora of complementary therapies brought temporary relief. But 18 years on I was still living within a circle of negativity no nearer to finding the cause of the illness to break the cycle.

In May 2003 I read a newspaper article about Mickel Therapy and booked for a course of treatment at the Edinburgh clinic.

My therapist was sympathetic and understanding and gave this drug-free therapeutic programme to work with that changed my whole perspective of the illness. Miraculously a door of hope was opened for me.

6 months following my initial treatment I am permanently cured and free of the ME.

Thank you Mickel Therapy for releasing me from this cycle of negativity.

DH-J 2004

Four years ago I thought I had everything. I was at university studying Physics in a city I loved, with good friends, a loving partner and a bright future. Within a year

I was unable to study, work or walk without help. I lost most of my friends because I couldn't go out, or they thought I was being lazy when I couldn't make plans to see them because I didn't know how I would be feeling. Many of them were sympathetic for the first couple of months, but then, when I didn't look sick and they couldn't tell what was really wrong with me, they began to get annoyed with me. Many of them told me that I just needed to think positively, or that I was wearing the illness as a label, or that I was just screwed up. I just needed to push myself a bit harder, do a little more every day, and not give in to it. The problem was that I thought that too. I thought I just needed to build up my strength and that I wasn't going to let it control my life. And so I got worse, and worse, and worse.

Over the next two years I lost the ability to read for more than a page at a time, I was confined to a wheelchair when outside the house and I needed a full-time carer. I couldn't cook, clean, walk or read. I couldn't wash myself without help, talk to anyone for longer than ten minutes without feeling drained or concentrate on anything for any length of time. Eventually I could do about ten or twenty minutes of activity a day and the rest of the time I just had to lie down somewhere dark. I felt like I was losing my mind as I watched all my dreams crumble.

Worst of all, no-one could give me any real help. I was shunted from doctor to doctor, many of whom were absolutely clueless, and some downright dangerous. I had one consultant launch a half-hour tirade about how evil I was for making everyone feel sorry for me so I never had to deal with anything or do anything for myself; that I was just manipulative and cruel; that ME groups were evil because it was in their interests to keep me sick and so they'd never give me any help. Although I lodged a complaint against him, it was never taken any further because I didn't have the energy to attend a tribunal.

I was on a cocktail of drugs for my myriad symptoms which included constant pain, nausea so bad that most days I could only eat one small meal and had to lie still for hours waiting for the feeling to subside, stiffness and dizziness. I had osteopathy, acupuncture, homeopathy and psychotherapy in addition to traditional medicine - all of which helped a bit but didn't cure me. And still I got worse. I had decided to kill myself if I got to the stage of being constantly bed-bound and incapable of anything for more than two months. It looked like I was headed that way, and so I had written letters to my family and close friends explaining my decision.

And then, one day, I got a phone call from my partner's father, saying that his mother had sent him an article from her local newspaper about a doctor who may have found a cure. Something clicked inside and, although I was sceptical after years of 'miracle cures' falling flat, I wanted to try it out. And so, for my 22nd birthday, my mother gave me the money for Mickel Therapy.

The journey to my first appointment exhausted me, and yet, when I came out I didn't feel as bad as I would normally have done. I even went home and talked to my mother for a while before I went to bed. I had the beginnings of hope, although I was terrified that I would be disappointed again. As I continued with the therapy I began to feel stronger and stronger. My muscle pain eased and my concentration came back. Although I still couldn't walk any real distance, I was able to use an electric wheelchair without getting confused and panicking.

After the second appointment I walked to the corner shop and back. It was a relatively tiny distance but was the furthest I had walked in three years. I was elated and terrified all at the same time. I was convinced it would go away again, that I would get sick again. Over the next few months, I began to walk more and more. I was able to go out to see my friends, some of whom cried at the sight of me walking again, with awareness in my eyes instead of clouds. One day I walked to the beach and back - a distance of a couple of miles. It took a long time and I had to rest on the way back, but I saw the sunrise over the water and knew that my life had changed. I was alive again.

At first I went out every night, saw my friends every day: scared that I would get sick again and so I was going to get as much use out of this remission as I could. But as the months went on, it didn't come back. I began to look at getting a part-time job, and fell in love again. Nearly a year after starting the therapy, I have just had my sixth appointment, have just bought a flat, am volunteering at a charity shop, have a great partner who is moving in with me and I have dreams for the future again. I am overwhelmed with possibility, but now that I know my health is here to stay, I am able to take my time to decide what I want to do. It was definitely the best birthday present I have ever been given.

FB - 2003

Appendix

Contact Details

Via website – www.mickeltherapy.com

E-mail - info@mickeltherapy.com

Telephone number – 01343831013
(answer machine service)

By Post – Mickel Health Initiatives Ltd
PO Box 6707
Elgin IV30 5WZ
Scotland